Lose The Emotional Baggage: Transform Your Mind & Spirit with Fasting

How to Lose Weight Fast and Renew the Mind, Body & Spirit with Fasting, Smart Eating and Practical Spirituality - Volume 5

I0419912

ROBERT DAVE JOHNSTON

Published by:

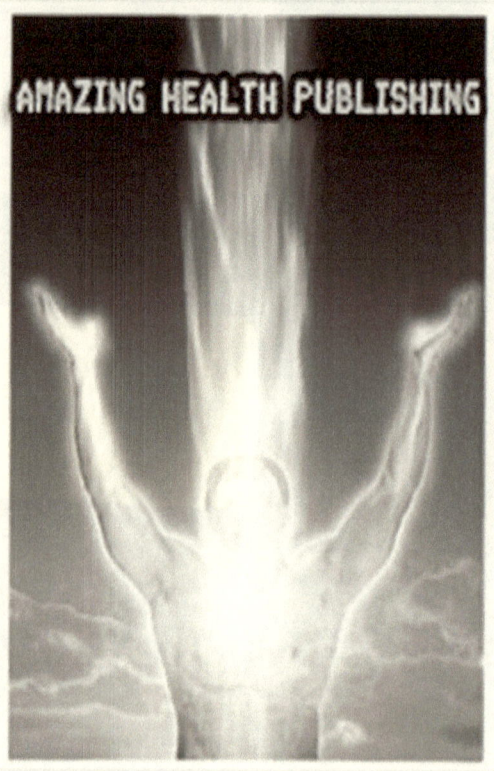

Follow Rob on Twitter @FitnessFasting

Copyright

Disclaimer & Legal Notices

The health-related information and suggestions contained in any of the books or written material mentioned above are based on the research, experience and opinions of the Author and other contributors. Nothing herein should be misinterpreted as actual medical advice, such as one would obtain from a Physician, or as advice for self-diagnosis or as any manner of prescription for self-treatment.

Neither is any information herein to be considered a particular or general cure for any ailment, disease or other health issue. The material contained within is offered strictly and solely for the purpose of providing Holistic health education to the general public. Persons with any health condition should consult a medical professional before entering this or any fasting, weight loss, detoxification or health related program.

Even if you suffer from no known illness, we recommend that you seek medical advice before starting any fasting, weight loss and/or detoxification program, and before choosing to follow any advice given this book. For any products or services mentioned or suggested in this book, you should read all packaging and instructions, as no substance, natural or drug, can be guaranteed to work in everyone.

Information and statements regarding dietary supplements, products or services mentioned in this book many not have been evaluated by the Food and Drug Administration and are not intended to diagnose, treat, cure, or prevent any disease. Never disregard or delay in seeking professional medical advice because of something you have read in this book.

Nothing that you read in this book should be regarded as medical or health advice. If you do anything recommended in this book, without the supervision of a licensed medical doctor, you do so at your own risk. Not recommended for persons with any health related condition unless supervised by a qualified health practitioner.

Because there is always some risk involved in any health-related program, the Author, Publisher and contributors assume no responsibility for any adverse effects or consequences resulting from the use of any suggested preparations or procedures described in any of the books or other written materials associated with the website FitnessThroughFasting.com. The author reserves the right to alter and update his opinions based on new conditions at any time.

Dedication

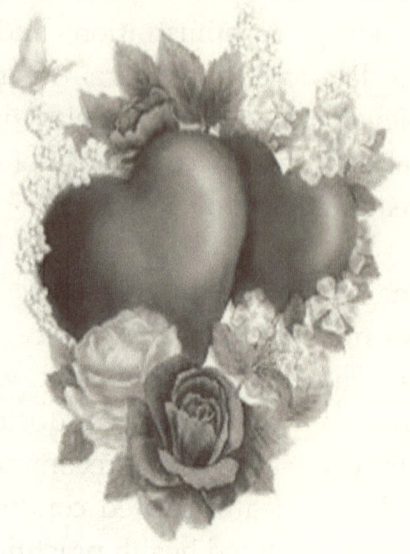

This series of books are dedicated to my mother Sonia Noemi, without whom I would not even be alive today. I love you mom. Thank you for never losing faith in me and supporting me, even when everything seemed hopeless and everyone else had given up on me. I owe you everything. I could collect all of the precious stones on this earth and lay them on your lap, and even still, I would not even come close to giving back to you all that you have given me.

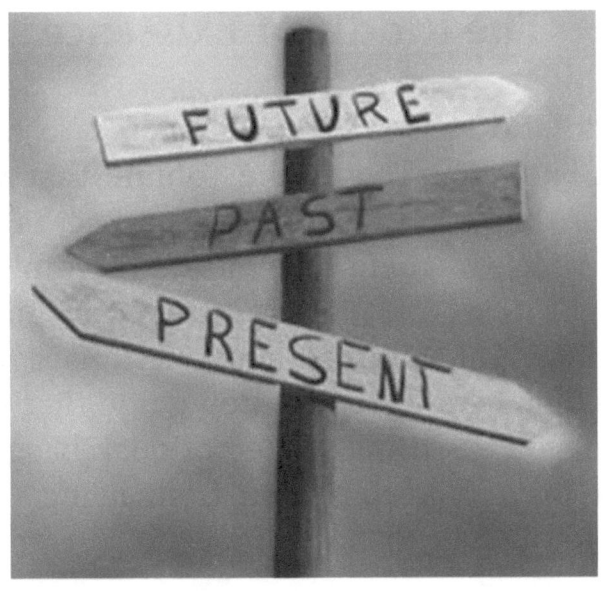

People write me and often ask: *"What's the point of life anyway? Why shouldn't I just end it all and stop this suffering?"* My response is usually the same: *"The point of it all is to keep fighting, seeking and moving forward until we achieve our breakthrough. If you choose to 'end it all,' many who would have benefited from your experience will be left behind without the hope and light that you were supposed to give them."*

Chapter 1:
The Riddle of Existence

Hello and welcome. I am honored to have you with me. This is the volume that will cover the *practical spirituality* aspect of the series. We're going to set aside the topic of weight loss and focus instead on inner healing and spiritual matters. I have put together here a step-by-step guide that will help you to drop the emotional baggage that may be keeping you from living your life to the fullest.

I will get into some deep waters here, and you may initially wonder what the heck this is all about. But I ask you to stick with me and take your time reading the material. Some of what I will ask you to do may initially seem off-the-wall. Get over it and do it anyways. This is the very system that I used years ago when I was stuck in a terrible cycle of depression, self-hatred, suicidal ideation, isolation and bitterness. It was the worst place that any human being could be in.

The formula that I share with you here was presented to me by one of my first mentors,

John Benitez, may he rest in peace - my precious and beautiful brother in arms. I miss him with every fiber of my heart. What courage he had!

Even though he had only one leg and had to overcome crippling addictions and behavior problems, he had gone on to become one of the most beautiful human beings that I have ever met. This book is a testament of his work because, without him, I am sure that I would either be dead or locked in some apartment gorging and killing myself.

This stuff is powerful and will help you a lot. If you have been struggling with internal wounds, memories, painful emotions, belief systems and behaviors that keep you from living and enjoying your life, then you are in the right place. I am not God, I don't have a crystal ball or have any mental powers... so I cannot tell you: *"I know that **FOR SURE** you are going to receive immediate healing."* If I came around giving guarantees I'd be a quack and not worthy of consideration.

However, I do want to tell you that, if you are honest and do the work to the best of your ability, then you are on your way to amazing changes in your life. People from all walks of life have escaped years of emotional bondage through prayer and fasting.

When I say prayer, I do not use the word in a religious, repetitive fashion. Prayer, to me, is simply having a conversation with the God of my understanding. Communicating my thoughts, feelings as well as asking for strength, help, guidance, protection and deliverance. The reason I make this clarification is because people have written me to ask if it was possible for them to receive spiritual benefit from fasting if they weren't Catholic, Christian, Buddhist or part of some other religion.

My answer is **ABSOLUTELY**. No religion is required to benefit from the power of prayer and fasting. All that is needed is a sincere willingness to seek for the answers. In addition to talking about prayer and fasting, this book will also present a **TEN-STEP** process that I call **The Ultimate Freedom Formula**. In it, you will do some heavy-duty introspection and house cleaning. The aim is to rid the soul of all of the rot that has been there for years causing you pain.

And I know all about rot and pain because I lived in it for more than 20 years.

My Personal Hell

Here's a sneak peek of where I come from: About 12 years ago I was 110 pounds overweight and completely taken over by chronic binge eating. It was not unusual for me to wake up in my living room floor covered in urine and vomit and surrounded by empty beer cans, pizza boxes and countless take-out bags from every restaurant under the sun.

I believed that I was trash and I treated myself as such. I was going to give God, the world and life my middle finger and keep eating until my stomach exploded and the whole craphouse went down in flames.

That was exactly my plan. I was filled with hatred, bitterness, sadness and rage. The emptiness that I lived in was like a bottomless black hole. There was nothing there except death and blackness. If you can visualize the condition that I was in, the complete loss of all human dignity ... that was my bottom. And yet, today, I am free of that emotional onslaught, and I have slimed down to my lowest weight ever at 205 pounds. More importantly, all of that emotional filth has pretty much vanished. I go through the normal ups and downs of existence, but that demon that kept sinking its teeth into my soul is gone. Whatever your 'demon' may be... it, too, is about to be tossed out on his *arse*.

The time has arrived for your healing to materialize and for you to step into the life that you have always dreamed. I believe with all of my heart that you will receive this healing, and I am putting my entire being into this book so you can feel that I care and love you. As a fellow traveler, we are kindred spirits and, while our lives may differ in many ways, our goals right now are the same - to receive emotional healing and personal transformation.

And there is **NOTHING** that the power of God cannot accomplish. Add fasting and faith into the mix, and what you have is a supernova explosion of healing and restoration. So no matter how bad you think your situation may be, the same power that touched me is available for you. I know that it works, not just because it did for me, but because I have had the privilege of corresponding with (*and meeting*) others who have traveled the path.

One friend that I will call Ronnie was raped repeatedly by her own father and brothers. They were involved in Satanism and offered her to 'the devil.' She was beaten to a pulp and raped over and over for years. Another friend I will call William was only nine when he was locked in a closet and forced to stay there for 10 to 18 hours at a time with no food or water. The abuse went on for five years until a neighbor called children services. William was removed from his parents' care and spent the next 10 years is foster care and juvenile detention facilities.

Drug addiction, alcoholism, gambling, adultery, eating disorders, chronic depression, suicide attempts, mental illness, post-traumatic stress disorder... whatever may be causing you pain ... it also can be healed and restored. In spite of the horrendous abuse she suffered, my friend Ronnie is vibrant today, full of joy and laughter.

William is happily married and has a beautiful daughter. He's always laughing and joking around. I say all of this to you because I want you to put to rest any doubt you may have about your own breakthrough. If it has happened for people like me and my friends, then it also will come to pass for you. Your life is **NOT** over. **The best is yet to come**!

The Reason for Living

What exactly is the healing that you seek? There may be issues in your life that you wish to resolve, wounds that you want to heal. Perhaps there are belief systems that constantly tell you that you are no good, that your life will never amount to anything.

Maybe you have given up. Perhaps despair, depression and hopelessness have become regular companions. Many people who visit my website **FitnessThroughFasting.com** write me with these very same challenges. They ask me: *"What's the point of life anyway? Why shouldn't I just end it all and stop this suffering?"* My response is usually the same: *"The point of it all is to keep fighting, seeking and moving forward until* *we achieve our breakthrough. If you choose to 'end it all,' many who would have benefited from your experience will be left behind without the hope and light that you were supposed to give them. And what about the possibilities for your own life? How do you know that, starting tomorrow, everything cannot change and you can move to a phase of ultimate freedom and happiness? Are you truly prepared to quit before the miracle happens?"*

That sounds well and fine. But what are we to do when hope and light seem to have totally vanished? When, no matter how hard we try, life still doesn't make sense or fall into place?

One lady that I spoke to recently told me that she felt as if an invisible butcher's knife was always stuck in her heart. That the emotional pain never went away. That she had prayed, prayed and prayed... she had gone to psychologists, taken medications and even undergone an exorcism, but - she indicated - the pain continued without any relief in sight. My heart went out to here because I knew exactly what she was talking about.

I have struggled with depression my whole life. What about you? Do you go through long periods of sadness and emotional pain? My question to you right now is: What would have to happen in order for you to feel <u>really</u> free? I am not talking about money or anything external. I mean, what would have to happen **IN YOUR HEART AND SOUL** for you to feel joy again?

Getting Additional Help

Note: This book presents a spiritual and practical plan for inner healing and restoration. However, if you are suffering from severe depression, have thoughts of suicide or of harming someone else, please seek professional help immediately.

Do not by any means substitute this book for treatment with a qualified mental health professional. Do not stop taking any mental health medications unless so indicated by your doctor. I know that using meds can be a drag and you may wish to be free of them. **But everything in its due time**... let's proceed with determination but also with caution.

Moreover, I want you to know that, apart from fasting, I also work regularly with a therapist who monitors my moods and helps me when I struggle. I am not superman or a 'special' being immune to human afflictions. I need to take care of myself and practice everything that I share with you.

Here's my point: I don't want you to enter into this thinking that **ALL** you have to do is follow this program and all will be fixed. I am not a doctor or a therapist, and it would be wrong for me to make such claims. In fact, I strongly urge you to find a good therapist in your area so that you can press on with your healing and spiritual growth once your work here is completed. **Don't try to go at this alone.**

Make sure that you have at least **ONE** person close to you that knows what you intend to do and supports you. At any rate, part of our work together involves that very person. So make sure to choose who he or she is going to be. It is usually better if this person is **NOT** directly related to you. If you have a best friend, then that is the best option.

We need somebody who will be supportive and not judgmental. **<u>Bottom line</u>**: There aren't any lone rangers in mental/emotional health. We need to stick together and help one another. Here's what I **<u>CAN</u>** tell you: The kind of practical spiritual work that we will do here, when done with honesty and a <u>real</u> desire to change, will have a remarkable impact on your mind, emotions and overall view of life, others and the world. Most of all, it will help you to start looking at yourself in a brand new light. One of hope and freedom!

The Journal

We are going to be asking ourselves a lot of questions. Also, there are many things that I want you to start to think and write about. For that reason, one of the most important tools that you'll need is a journal. Not a junk notebook full of scribbles and other notes. I want you to go out and purchase a special *'Healing Journal,'* a place where you can jot down your inmost thoughts and feelings.

Later in the book I'll be asking you to do some thorough internal work. And we'll need a journal to get the job done.

Before you go any further, make sure that you have this all-important item. If you already have one, then continue to use it, although I encourage you to purchase a new one so we can start *'fresh.'* From now on, I am going to assume that you have the journal and I'll be asking you to write your thoughts on a variety of subjects. So let's get to it!

Chapter 2:
The Path to
Healing & Renewal

Maybe there has been abuse in your past. There definitely was in mine. When I first started fasting, in a rare type of epiphany, I suddenly recalled being molested when I was 8 years old. Nothing special happened at that particular moment to elicit those hidden memories. They just appeared in my conscious mind. "Boom!" There it was...just like that.

I couldn't remember who the person was that molested me, but the memory of the act was quite clear. Ugly, sickening stuff. I dare to be transparent with you because I have made my peace. I can share it with you with my head held high because I no longer blame myself or anybody else. What happened, happened. I refuse to continue to flog myself for the mistakes of others. And it was through fasting and following the process that I am going to share with you here that I made strides toward recovery. It is my faith and hope that you, too, will experience the same restoration.

In one way or another, we've all been damaged. No human being on this earth is immune to pain and suffering. But that doesn't mean that we should allow the wounds to fester. No matter what we may have gone through in the past, we **MUST** persevere and continue to believe. Believe even when it appears that there's nothing left to believe in. Rekindling that belief is what this book is all about... the belief in life... the belief in goodness ... **the belief in yourself**.

Prayer and Fasting

We are coming together to tap into a mystery. A mystery that opens steel doors and gates of bronze. A mystery that works when other methods do not. When Jesus' apostles were unable to heal a man from his sickness (*which is said to have been demonic possession*), they went to the Master and asked Him for help.

Once Jesus had healed the man, the apostles asked Him why He was able to do it but they weren't. Jesus told them: "*This kind only comes out through prayer and fasting.*" **Mark 9:27:-29.**

What did Jesus mean by this? This question is the source of much debate. Some say Jesus was talking about high-ranking demonic spirits that could only be defeated by the increased spiritual authority attained through prayer combined with fasting.

Others refute the demon argument, indicating that Jesus was referring to the apostles' spiritual immaturity. In my opinion, through that statement, Jesus gave the apostles a powerful clue as to **how the spiritual world operates**. Let me share this analogy to illustrate: A man who has never gone to the gym will need to work hard and long to be able to lift 300 pounds, right?

Likewise, as beings attached to the physical world, we must work consistently to overcome the veil of illusion (*world of matter and appearances*) and enter more-fully into the spirit world. In other words, **I believe that the miracles that you seek have already happened. Now it is your job to grow spiritually until you break through the fear, doubt and unbelief that keeps you from believing, seeing and receiving it.**

And nothing breaks through the stubborn walls of the ego as effectively and thoroughly as fasting.

This means that the struggles, abuses and emotional wounds you've suffered now have become the roadmap to your destiny and spiritual awakening. After all, if you did not feel the need for healing and breakthrough, why would you be reading this book? Is it not the very pain that we feel which propels us to seek for answers? **Where is the incentive to pray, fast and grow spiritually if everything is sunshine and rainbows?** Perhaps one could say that curiosity would lead one to seek for the answers. But the truth is that **PAIN IS THE GREATEST OF ALL MOTIVATORS**.

When we are in enough pain, we become willing to set aside prejudice, apathy and doubt. Pain has a way of beating us into submission. And I understand you because I myself come from the same path. Together we can walk towards a tangible solution.

All I ask is that you remain open-minded and do the work I present to the very best of your ability.

Special Note: I want this book to be all-inclusive. In other words, whether you have strong religious beliefs or not, you still have a place in this work. Even though I myself am a Christian, if your beliefs are different and belong to another creed, you are still very much welcome. **Here there is no division**.

Rather, we will focus on that which <u>brings us togeth</u>er. And that is our humanity, as well as our quest to transcend what limits us. Regardless of our skin color, background, creed or social status, we now come together as one. And, ironically, it is by leaving behind prejudice and division that we are able to find ourselves and fulfill our life's purpose.

Now let's look at the role that fasting plays in this process of healing and awakening.

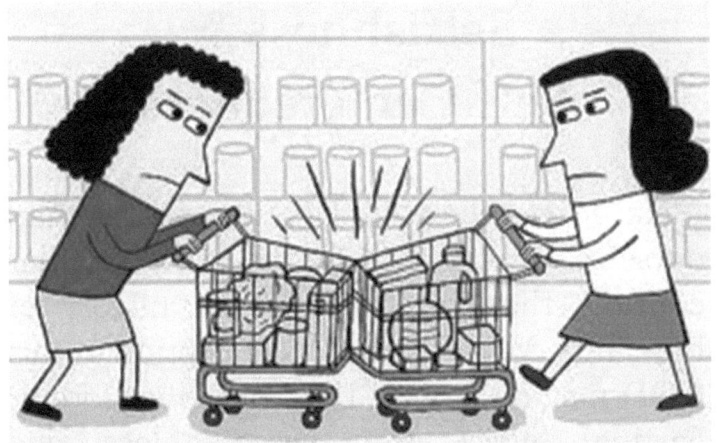

"Selfishness, self-centeredness are the primary culprits in all human conflict Most people live life through *"self-propulsion"*, eating, sleeping, working, striving, controlling and forever fighting to craft their lives according to their own designs."

Chapter 3:
Selfishness &
Self-Centeredness

Most of us believe in a Power greater than ourselves... a Czar of the universe that controls the heavens and the history of humanity. Whatever your conception of this **GOD** may be, now is the time to explore it. Fasting (*apart from weight loss and detoxification*) has the "secondary effect" of removing our attention from physical appetites and placing it in **the higher realm of God, Life and Existence**. Here's the thing: Food truly controls humanity. *"When do we eat? What do we eat? I am hungry!" These are all statements that (usually) are more common than: "Who am I? Why am I here? What is the purpose of my life?"*

Aren't most of us primarily concerned with our bodies, our appetites and our bellies? Today's society is *"externally-oriented"*. In other words, it is all about the body, the looks, the material possessions ... **me, me, me!** It's all about me!

Have you ever put on the turn signal in your car to change lanes in high traffic? What usually happens? Are you given right-of-way? Or do you find that most cars speed up to keep you from passing? Sadly, in the majority of cases, it is the latter. So what is the problem? **Selfishness, self-centeredness, that is the problem**! Most people live life through *"self-propulsion"*, eating, sleeping, working, striving, controlling and forever fighting to craft their lives according to their own designs.

When fasting, one is able to withdraw from the self-centered masses long enough to wonder:

"...there has to be more out there than just me, my limited thinking and what I think life should be. There has got to be some type of Higher Power... God - an ultimate being that knows better than me and has the ability to help me with my life and show me which way I should go".

When we fast, we begin to see just how limited we are in our humanity. We start to realize that our understanding of life and existence is superficial at best.

Could it be that self-propulsion, human wisdom and strength are insufficient to carry us through life? Is it possible that by growing spiritually we can <u>gain insight and have a greater understanding of our lives; finding peace within</u>? What about the daily trials we go through? That situation which, no matter what we do, does not seem to budge:

Is Divine Intervention possible?

And what of that illness? Can it heal? What if we come to find out that we don't know who we really are? What if the reason for your existence has yet to be fully revealed? Can fasting lead us to the answer? My answer is: yes and yes. But the biggest question I recall asking myself was: Who is God?

Chapter 4:
Who is God?

God has been described as everything from an impersonal life-force to a benevolent, personal, almighty Creator embodied in His Son Jesus Christ. The figure of God has also been called by many other names, including: Zeus, Jupiter, Brahma, Allah, Ra, Odin, Ashur, Izanagi, Viracocha, Ahura Mazda, and The Great Spirit (*Wakan Tanka*) to name just a few. God is seen by some simply as Mother Nature and by others as Father God, Father Sky and Mother Goddess. But who is God really?

What is <u>YOUR</u> specific concept of God? Where did this concept come from? Childhood? Your own studies? How has this belief impacted your life? Has it made a difference? If yes, how so? Take some time and write these questions in your journal and answer them to the very best of your ability. Perhaps you are confused with this "God thing." Is there even a God? If God is real, why have so many bad things happened? Can I trust God?

Take the time and work at answering all of these questions. Learning what God's attributes are helped me to start moving towards some understanding. Let's take a look...

God's Divine Attributes

Here are some key characteristics associated with the Christian God.

Infinite: God knows no boundaries. He is without measure. This attribute by definition impacts all of the others. Since God is infinite, everything else about Him must also be infinite. God lives above time ... the past, present and future are **ALL** under His direct control.

Wisdom: Wisdom is the ability to devise perfect ends and to achieve these ends by the most perfect means. In other words, God makes no mistakes.

Omniscient: God possesses perfect knowledge and, consequently, has no need to learn anything. God has never learned and cannot learn because he has always known everything.

Omniscience means all-knowing. God knows everything, and His knowledge is infinite. It is impossible to hide anything from God because, in essence, He knows that you are going to do before you even do it.

Omnipotent: Literally, this word means all-powerful. Since God is infinite and, since He possesses all knowledge, then His power is absolute and indivisible. Nothing is more powerful than God. God cannot be defeated or overpowered. He allows us to partake in His power, but the source is always Him. All things are possible for God. Nothing is beyond God's ability to accomplish.

Sovereign: God is above all creation and is the absolute and ultimate ruler of the universes. Nothing is higher than God. Since He knows everything and can do anything, he alone controls all things, weighs all things and holds the history of mankind in the palm of His hand. Being sovereign gives God total freedom to do as he sees fit in all things. In spite of this, human beings have the power of choice and will always have to face the consequences of our actions.

God's sovereignty does not remove will power from humans.

Self-Existent: When Moses asked who he was talking to in the burning bush, God said, *"I AM THAT I AM"* God has no beginning or end. He just exists. Nothing else in the entire universe is self-caused. Only God. In fact, if anything else had created Him, that thing would be God. This is a difficult concept for our minds since everything we encounter comes from something other than itself. **God has always existed.**

Love: Love is such an important part of God's character that the apostle John wrote, *"God is love."* This means that God holds the well-being of others as His primary concern. For a full definition of love, read *1 Corinthians 13.* God's love is not a love of emotion but of action. His love gives freely to the object of its affection, his human creation. But we must open our minds and hearts to receive this love because God always respects our free will. He will never force Himself into our lives if He isn't invited.

To me, **that last attribute of love was difficult**. I was raised with the conception of a judging God with a beard - sitting on the clouds combing his long white hair, looking down at the earth and <u>always ready to throw lightning bolts at me for the slightest infraction</u>. This belief kept my spirituality dead for many years because, since I had fallen so far and low, I didn't consider myself worthy to receive His help. But, as it turns out, He was always there, with His arms wide open, waiting to receive and restore me.

Chapter 5:
The Question of
Evil & Suffering

One of the biggest stumbling blocks that I had in my spiritual path was:

"Well, if God is so great and full of love, why does he allow children to suffer, be raped and killed, why does he allow evil to win over good and why does everything seem to be going from bad to worse? Why do good people constantly suffer while the evil prosper?"

These are difficult questions that troubled me deeply for years. The only answer that I have is: I don't know. Honestly, there is **NO** explanation that satisfies me fully. There is the premise that, as humans, we see and comprehend only as far as our dimensional existence allows us to.

Therefore, we are unable to fully grasp God's *'super-human'* thoughts, intentions and plans. I admit that, as humans, there are many things about God which we won't understand.

Just as an ant will never be able to understand New York City, so is *'the mind of God'* an enigma to the human intellect.

However, to me... there had to be a more satisfactory answer. **And the one I have found is this:** If you want suffering to be reduced in the world around you, then <u>you must become an agent of healing and change</u>. If I sit around in my own crap and do nothing to improve the quality of my life, then I am adding to the suffering and contributing nothing to the healing. I become part of the problem. The best way to heal the world is to **start by healing yourself**.

Then you'll be able to share the healing with everyone around you and make the light grow bigger. God can use your arms, legs and mind to do **<u>A LOT</u>** of good in this world. **What I want to say to you is this**:

Do not allow the *'questions'* of existence to stop you from pressing forward toward your <u>healing and restoration</u>. Whatever answers you don't have **<u>NOW</u>** will come **<u>LATER</u>** as you progress spiritually.

New questions will certainly emerge as you go forward. And those, too, will be answered in their own time.

Emotional Quicksand

To allow ourselves to get stuck in the 'whys' is tragic because we remain immobilized... trapped in emotional quicksand. Throw away the thought that "unless I can understand why God does this and that... then I can never believe." **Nobody is asking you to believe anything**. I certainly am not here to fill you with any dogma, or to convince you to believe anything.

All you need is to become "willing to believe that 'maybe' there is 'something out there' that can help me." If you can simply 'crack the door' of your mind open and leave it ajar, just a tiny bit, then **that is more than enough to begin**. A small amount of willingness to believe that 'maybe' this can happen will allow the light of possibility to get through. And that is sufficient to get the ball rolling.

Chapter 6:
The Transforming
Power of Fasting

Fasting on a regular basis has been the key to my physical and emotional healing. Without fasting, I'd still be plagued with depression, bitterness, fear, isolation, suicidal ideation, hopelessness etc... Fasting helped me to heal faster because it led me to place greater emphasis on spiritual growth.

Fasting put me face-to-face with all of the negativity and emotional pain that tormented me. **Being able to face and process this pain has allowed my spirit to grow**. Today my job is to remain vigilant and quickly uproot and throw away the mental weeds that try to break the surface. Where there used to be only fear and unbelief, now there's faith and hope.

What I mean is this: Without fasting, the negative emotions and belief systems controlled my thoughts, emotions and behaviors. They were very painful to resist. My heart and soul were weak and beaten.

All I could do was sit in a corner taking blows, 'hoping' that it would stop. **I had no willingness to fight because I thought that freedom was impossible**. Fasting changed all of that by giving my spirit a shot of *'spiritual spinach.'* And. like Popeye, I was able to rise and fight against the internal bullies that wanted to keep me down.

I experienced a <u>profound physical, mental and spiritual revolution</u>. If you can believe that God has the attributes that we talked about in the previous chapter, then the truth is clear: There is **<u>NOTHING</u>** that can't be transformed, refreshed and/or healed through the spiritual power one gains with fasting. Many who visit my main website **FitnessThroughFasting.com** write me and ask: *"Why is fasting a doorway to spirituality"* Fasting can alter the course of your life and lead you to unprecedented levels of health, inner peace and vitality. It did for me!

Fasting gets our minds away from constant preoccupation with the external needs of the body and makes us more sensitive to the internal world of thought, emotion and spirit.

It unearths many memories, feelings, ideas, beliefs and perceptions that we weren't completely aware of. And this constant suppression of our inner world is, by far, one of the biggest causes of spiritual sickness.

Signs of Spiritual Sickness

* A sudden onset of apathy or listlessness.
* Lack of initiative or enthusiasm.
* Lack of joy.
* Blocked memory: Inability to remember parts of one's life.
* Inability to feel love or receive love from another.
* Emotional remoteness.
* Failure to thrive.
* Inability to make decisions.
* Chronic negativity.
* Addictions.
* Suicidal Tendencies
* Constant Melancholy or despair.
* Chronic depression.
* Loss of desire to live

Please take a moment and go through each of the symptoms above.

How many of them were you able to identify in your own life?

At one point, I could say 'yes' to all of them. Do only one or two pertain to you, or do you find that you can relate to many (*if not all*) of them? We are simply evaluating ourselves here. Please do not judge or put any other negative charge into what we are doing. Let's look at the list simply as a measuring instrument. Read each one of the symptoms listed. Pause and think. Which ones have given you the most trouble in the past year? How so? Write about it in your journal.

After going through the list, what is your conclusion? Would you say that you are spiritually sick? Only you can diagnose yourself. /Be honest and thorough in your assessment.

What have you discovered from going through the list?

How bad would you say is your condition? Whatever the case may be... please don't put yourself down. You have taken the time to buy this book because you want to be part of the solution, right? Give yourself credit for that.

Looking Inward

The answers are within and waiting to be seized. But getting in touch with the spiritual is challenging because we live in a material and superficial world. That is why fasting is so powerful. It gives us the opportunity to reconnect with our minds and bodies in a more personal and quiet way.

Fasting increases self-awareness, self-control, self-restraint and patience. We become more attuned to introspection and are thus able to see ourselves with detached objectivity.

It helps us to *"get out of our own way."* As the protective layer of **EGO** yields, we start to feel *(and release)* old memories, thoughts and emotions. This release is crucial because it gives us deeper insight into ourselves. Many have described the process as going into *"the unknown,"* a huge break from their old, established ways of being.

During a fast, your body and mind get to unwind from stress. The deeper spiritual dimension, on the other hand, comes alive and is brought to the forefront of our awareness.

As the fast continues, a profound sense of peace and serenity wells up, **like a constant meditation is taking place within you**. You will feel a fresh and powerful connection with your *'core'* being... the part of you connected directly to the spiritual.

This sense of surrender profoundly heightens our spiritual connection.

And that connection is the one that has the healing power that you're looking for. That spiritual connection is the one that will purge the painful and negative belief systems that have hurt you. So let's continue moving forward with the task at hand.

Chapter 7:
Types of Fasting

Before we enter into the actual inner work, there are <u>two key questions</u> that I need you to answer. Those are: **A**-What type of fasting will you do? **B**- For how long will you fast? To help you decide, let's look at the various '*types*' of fasting practices available. I will make my personal recommendation at the end. Still, I want you to have all of the information here in front of you. Ultimately, you can decide for yourself which path you wish to follow. I will make it as simple and painless as possible and guide you step by step. <u>**Quick note**</u>: To get a <u>**LOT**</u> more detail about juice fasting and intermittent fasting, I encourage you to read **Volumes 2 and 5** of this series, respectively.

Water Fasting is considered the purest form of fasting. It involves **going a period of time without eating, drinking only water.** Weight loss while water fasting ranges from 1 to 20 pounds (*or more*) in the first seven days. After that, the body (*commonly*) settles into a fat-burning '*pace*' of **one-to-three pounds per day**.

Specific weight loss figures will depend on how the body responds, as well as a person's overall state of health. Twenty to 30% of the <u>initial</u> weight lost with water fasting is water weight, <u>not fat</u>. Once the longer-term pace is reached, water weight loss diminishes. At that point the body will 'eat' one-to-three pounds of pure fat daily. Again, these numbers fluctuate according to a person's body makeup and general health.

Absolute Fasting. (*also known as dry fasting*) is the hardest and strictest form of fasting. It entails going a period of time (*no more than 72 hours are recommended*) without eating **OR** drinking liquids of any kind. There are two kinds of absolute fasting: *soft and dry*. Soft dry fasting allows 'external' contact with water as taking a shower, going swimming etc.

With <u>hard</u> dry fasting, the practitioner abstains from **ALL** contact with water, even showering. Dry fasting produces the fastest and most dramatic weight loss, approximately 20 pounds in three days. Most of the weight loss, however, is comprised of water weight because the body goes into dehydration.

There are some who maintain that absolute fasting could cure the common cold if practiced when symptoms first emerge. I have read cases of people who have done an absolute fast for three-to-five days and were reportedly cured of life-long allergic reactions and conditions. The process behind the healing power of dry fasting is that, since the body is not receiving food or hydration, overall bodily functions slow to a minimum. Consequently, it is believed, the immune system has a much greater amount of resources to seek and destroy all sort of sickness - even viruses.

While with juice and water fasting bodily functions slow down considerably, **a dry fast reduces them much further**. This deeper reduction in body functions, it is believed, gives the immune system ultra-healing capacity. Sort of like having been stuck in a traffic jam and then, suddenly, having the entire interstate all to yourself. You don't have to share the highway any longer. Therefore, you can step on the gas freely because <u>the traffic with which you were sharing the road is no longer there</u>. I completed a 72-hour dry fast some years ago and can tell you that it is probably among the hardest things I've ever done. You can read more about my dry fasting experience at the main website **FitnessThroughFasting.com**. Dry fasting is dangerous and should not be practiced unless one is **<u>VERY</u>** experienced in fasting and calorie restriction.

Juice Fasting. is the most popular kind of fasting. It is a time during which one ingests only water as well as the juice from liquefied fruits and vegetables. My personal recipe is that of celery, tomatoes, broccoli, watercress, apples, pears, strawberries and blueberries - the liquid mixed in a gallon-jug and topped with water. I use this mixture regularly to do three and seven-day spurts of juice fasting.

So that is a very doable option for you. Juice fasting is popular because it is not as harsh as water or dry fasting. Rather than relying only on water, it pumps the body full of amazing nutrients. Overall, weight loss with juice fasting in the first 10 days can fluctuate from 7 to 20 pounds (*depending on health and body makeup*), and then settles on one-to-two pounds per day.

Which Type of Fast Should I Do?

If you are a beginner and have **NEVER** done any type of fasting, then I would recommend that you start with juice fasting. To make matters ultra-easy, I would suggest that you purchase some fresh fruit and veggie juice and use that for your fast. If you want to **REALLY** get into juicing and combining fruits and veggies, I would highly recommend that you check out the other book of the series **How to Lose 30 Pounds (Or More) In 30 Days With Juice Fasting**. There, I go step-by-step through the juicing recipe, the juicing process and basically lay it all out in detail.

But, for starters, you can do very well with juice that you purchase. You have to make sure that it is **NOT** commercial juice packed with sugar.

Get the healthiest and freshest type of juice that you can. I like the **Bolthouse Farms** brand and sometimes use it when I do short fasts of one-to-three days. But their fruit juices tend to have a lot of sugar.

I strongly recommend that you **combine fruit and veggie juice in a jar and then add water until the excessive sweetness is reduced.**

How Much Juice Do I Drink?

IF you are new to juice fasting, the key is to: <u>**KEEP IT SIMPLE**</u>. You are fasting for internal/spiritual purposes... the taste and mixture that you use is secondary. Of course, you want to have something to drink that you enjoy.

So find a mixture of fresh fruit and veggie juice that you can live with. But do not become overly preoccupied with the taste and ingredients of the juice at this point. I want your focus to be on your internal world, not on what the taste buds have to say about this or that juice.

In terms of daily juice amounts, you can drink **an eight-to-twelve-ounce of the juice every four hours, not exceeding 64 ounces of juice per day**. In addition to the juice, you must strive to drink at least one gallon of water daily.

To help with hunger and detox symptoms, use decaffeinated green tea, chamomile tea and seltzer water (*sparkling water/club soda*). These tools will go a long ways to calm you whenever there's any type of physical, mental or emotional disturbance.

One Gallon of Water Daily

If, on the other hand, you are experienced in fasting... then perhaps you are ready to do a straight water fast. Or maybe you don't have too much experience with fasting but have reached a point in your life where you are willing to sacrifice. If your choice is water fasting, then what matters most is - **QUALITY OF WATER**. Please avoid tap water at all costs. If you have a water purifier, then that is optimum. If not, then I advise you to boil the water that you are going to drink for at least five minutes. You should be drinking the purest water possible. **One gallon of water daily is the recipe.** And you can also use the decaf green tea, chamomile tea and seltzer water to help you navigate the rough spots.

I cannot recommend a dry fast. If what you are feeling in your heart is that you need to do a dry fast, then that is something that you must settle within your own conscience. When I did my three-day dry fast, it was a very personal adventure that I undertook because I wanted to pass along the information to others. But it is a very dangerous practice and should not be done lightly under any circumstances. Best if done with the direct supervision of a medical professional. Take a moment and evaluate the various options we've just looked at. Which type of fast have you decided to do? Write about your decision in your fasting journal.

For How Long Should I Fast?

Now you need to decide the length of the fast that you are going to do. I get into much more detail about intermittent fasting on <u>Volume 2</u> of this series titled **The Intermittent Fasting Weight Loss Formula**, so I encourage you to purchase and read that book as well when you have a chance. I also encourage you to check out <u>Volume 1</u> **The 'Permanent Weight Loss' Diet**. That book goes into great detail with dieting. It can help you to break the fast property and have a clean and solid diet to return to. I do not want for you to receive spiritual benefits from your fast, and then go back to a diet filled with refined sugar, flour and fatty foods. So please, it is very important that you realize that *'eating after fasting'* is even more important than fasting itself. I found that, **the cleaner and better I eat after each fast, the stronger the spiritual benefit I receive**. So I want you to think hard about your eating habits and, in addition to fasting, <u>make a commitment with yourself</u> to make permanent eating-habit changes once the fast is over.

So for how long should you fast? I myself did a 40-day water fast when I initially began my healing journey. *I was so beaten and emotionally destroyed that I had become willing to do <u>absolutely anything</u> to get better.* The pain had become so strong and overwhelming that going through fasting hunger and detox symptoms was no big deal. I even quit smoking cold turkey on the spot. I was a two-pack-a-day Marlboro Reds smoker, so that was in itself quite a miracle.

It all came down to willingness and being fed up of the way I was living my life.

Maybe you have reached the point where you can understand what I'm talking about. However, whatever the case may be: '*you do not have to break any fasting records to start receiving immediate benefit.*' If, right now, all that you are prepared to do is fast for 24 hours once weekly, then that is a good start. **Do what is within your grasp to do.** What matters is that you start to take action and not procrastinate.

My Recommendation

For the quickest push forward, I have found that **7-10 days of juice or water fasting will have tremendous impact spiritually and emotionally. Consider doing seven-to-ten full days of fasting at a very minimum**.

Look at it as a <u>spiritual investment</u> in the inner healing and growth and that you want to accomplish. You've eaten plenty in your life and, believe me, you shall eat again. Having a ten-day break is nothing horrible, and you certainly won't '*starve*' as some people think. Most people of average height and weight can actually go for at least 40 days without food **<u>BEFORE</u>** starvation begins. That number is even higher if the person is overweight. Some people cry the blues about *'having to go ten days without eating'* as if they were being asked to give up an arm or a leg. Their attachment to food is that strong. How about you?

How far are you willing to go? How important is it for you to receive healing and freedom in your life?

I encourage you to write these questions in your journal and answer them with as much gut-wrenching honesty as you can muster.

If, however, right now you simply cannot fast for that long, then I urge you to work towards it. Make it a goal to, at least once in your life, go through seven-to-10 days of juice or water fasting. Believe me, the experience is one that will stay with you for many years to come. It has the **potential to transform your life**.

However, there are some cases in which, due to illness or other reasons, fasting for seven days or more is simply not feasible. In that case, then make it a goal to do **THREE** full days of juice fasting or water fasting.

Bottom line: **Shoot for seven-to-ten days of juice or water fasting. If you are ill and cannot do this long, then opt for three days of juice or water fasting**.

If you still feel undecided, I invite you to visit the two fasting forums at **FitnessThroughFasting.com** and read through some of the posts. That way you can get a general idea of what others are doing and what makes you feel most comfortable. It's a good idea to start getting plugged in to these forums **BEFORE** you start the fast.

You will meet a lot of like-minded people. Then, when you begin to fast, you can go there anytime and receive ongoing support and encouragement. Just to be thorough, I have included below a list of some intermittent fasting alternatives that you can also consider, either for now or for future fasts.

Chapter 8:
Intermittent Fasting (IF)

As I said, not everyone may be ready to fast nonstop for days and days and days. However, there are shorter fasts that you can start to practice right way to build experience, strength and confidence. Let's take a look at what these options are:

Daily Intermittent Fasting: As in Catholic Lent Fasting and Muslim Ramadan, here you would fast from sunup to sundown - approximately <u>12 hours daily</u>. The fast is broken each night with a light meal, preferably lean fish or poultry, small portion of carbs (*4oz baked or sweet potato*) and steamed veggies. The *"eating window"* remains open until dawn. But for most of that time you will be sleeping.

Twelve hours to eat, twelve hours to fast... and so the cycle continues each day.

You can get up in the AM, have breakfast, and then fast for the next 12 hours. I love Daily (IF). It is great for beginners as well as the experienced because one can go with the daily fast for as long as desired. I know one person who fasted daily in this fashion for five years! Amazing... Estimated Weekly weight loss: <u>three to five pounds</u>.

Every Other Day Intermittent Fasting: Another form of intermittent fasting is to go for an entire 24-hour cycle every other day. <u>Example</u>: You fast from 8am Monday morning to 8am Tuesday morning. Eat lightly on Tuesday. Wake up on Wednesday at 7:30am and have breakfast. Start the fast at 8am until the same time on Thursday... and so on. Estimated Weekly weight loss: two to four pounds.

Half Week Intermittent Fasting: Fast for 3.5 days of the week. <u>Example</u>: Fast from 8am Monday to 8pm Thursday. You can return to regular eating for the rest of the week. **Fasting would resume the following Monday at 8am - repeating the same cycle**. This system requires caution, however. Since one does not eat for 84-hour periods, it will be necessary to follow the breaking a fast instructions, listed towards the end of this book. Estimated weekly weight loss: <u>three to five pounds</u>.

Seven Day Intermittent Fasting: Fast for an entire seven days, return to your regular diet for seven days, and then fast for another seven days. Similar to the Half Week method, you will need follow the breaking a fast instructions. Estimated weekly weight loss: <u>Five to 20 pounds during initial 7-day fast and five to seven on subsequent ones</u>.

Combination Intermittent Fasting: The ultimate way to practice intermittent fasting is to combine all of the above and complete 14 and 30-day cycles of intermittent fasts. Combination can also be doing 24-hour juice fasting once a week, three-day juice fasting weekly or bi-weekly... whatever is within your ability to do, **THAT** is more than enough to get started.

As I said already, what matters is that you jump aboard and get going. **By no means pressure yourself to do a long fast that you aren't mentally prepared to do.**

A lot of people that have fasted for 14 days and beyond first had to begin with shorter ones <u>to build their stamina</u>. So, if you are experienced and have done it before, then bon voyage - you're on your way. If, on the other hand, you are new to juice fasting, then do what you can and build from there. No matter what you are able to do, you come off a winner!

Make a Decision

Alright so now I want you to decide for how long you will be fasting. Weigh your options carefully, ponder on my recommendations and make a decision. We still have a lot of preparation to go through, so you can always come back later and re-evaluate your decision if need be.

However, right now I want you to go to your journal and place in writing **BOTH** the kind of fasting that you will do (*juice or water fasting*), **AND** the duration of the fast that you will start with. I say *'start with'* because I hope fasting is something that you continue to do **for the rest of your life.** It is a powerful practice, not only for spiritual and emotional growth, but also to keep the body lean and free of toxins. Studies in calorie-restriction and life-extension have proven that the less a human eats, the longer he or she tends to live.

So, to me, **fasting is about ultimate health, life and freedom.** And those are the three qualities that we are working towards in this book. Ok, so have you made your decision and written it down in your journal? Good. Make sure to write about the reasons why you are choosing this path right now. As time passes, <u>it will be very interesting for you to see where you were and how far you have come</u>. I have journals dating 10, 12 and 14 years that are absolute gems to me.

When I look back at my posts, my way of thinking and behaving, I can very much say that I have changed **<u>A LOT</u>**. And so will you. We all change. The point is *'changing for the better.'* Growing as a human being and rising to new challenges, **<u>NOT</u>** getting stuck in repeated/addictive behaviors and emotional wounds from the past.

Spend time in your journal daily writing your thoughts and feelings as you read this book. <u>Write freely and without restraint</u>. This journal is private, so what you write there is for your eyes only. Always keep it in a safe place, away from children or prying eyes.

Chapter 9:
Seizing the
Spiritual Potential

Now that you have decided the type of fast that you are going to do and for how long, it is time to start working on the *'inner foundation'* that will lead us to the breakthrough that we seek. And that foundation is based on what I call **"Five Steps to Seize the Spiritual Potential of Fasting."**

If you are ready to begin, then take out your fasting journal and let's get to work. Some of the things that I am going to ask you to do may feel silly at first. Ignore the negativity and continue to work. Identify that internal chatter that is always criticizing everything that you do and <u>tell it to shut up</u>!

1. Take a written inventory of everything *"external and/or physical"* that is going on in your life that you want to see change for the better. This can include health, finances, relationships, or anything else that is troubling you.

If there is an ongoing situation that is causing you stress, list it. Be thorough. When you are done, you should have a numbered list with a brief explanation of the negative feelings and/or consequences that each item causes. Then, in another brief sentence, write how you would feel to be free of that situation and how you would use that freedom for the benefit of others.

Example: "My binging: a) Causes me great guilt, shame and is harming me physically and keeping me from being more active and social. b) Being healed from binging would give me an amazing sense of freedom and make me a more effective person, both for my loved ones and others because I would lose weight, be healthier and more alive.

Tip: Notice that the key in the end is to write *"how being free of the situation will allow you to be of service to others"*.

How would being free of this internal baggage cause you to be more effective for the benefit of others? Example: Being free of these internal chains will cause me to be much more social and open to those who are suffering.

I could become a comforter and a motivator instead of someone who is always down and depressed. I could write books about my experience, start a website...etc...

2. Take a written inventory of everything "internal and/or emotional" that you want to change for the better. This often includes character defects that we identify in ourselves such as; shy, lazy, inconsistent, impatient, bitter, angry, depressed, hopeless, resentful etc... Next to each characteristic, list the negative effect that it is having in your life **AND** write the positive trait you would like to have instead. Conclude this step by writing a few brief sentences on how this emotional liberation would allow you to be a better person for the benefit of others.

<u>Example</u>: My depression: a) keeps me isolated from my friends, I don't want to see or talk to anybody and feel hopeless and dead on the inside. b) I want depression to be replaced with joy. Joy would allow me to see life through laughter and hope and I would be able to comfort others who are hurting by making them laugh or by giving them a lighter perspective.

3) Write a list of specific requests you have related to loved ones or friends that are hurting. Take stock of positive changes that you would like to see come to pass in the lives of the people around you. This can be the healing of a friend that is ill, comfort for a loved-one who is in mourning... anything that you want. There are no restrictions to these requests.

<u>Example</u>: **a**) My uncle: That he would find a job he enjoys and find some financial stability; **b**) My friend John and his wife: That they be able to work out their differences and save their marriage; **c**) My mother: That she be healed of her lower back and shoulder pains and that new opportunities emerge for her to practice her art;

d) My wife: That the doors to her profession be re-opened in a quality facility where she is appreciated and loved.

Notice that the request is that our loved ones and friends become better and more effective people.

4) This is the step where we come to realize our powerlessness. Look at everything that you have written in the first three steps and internalize the fact that you, of yourself, can do **NOTHING** to fix or rectify **ANY** of those items listed. When I first came to that realization, I was floored. You see, I was always the *"saver"*. I always wanted to take care of others and rescue them from their problems.

In the meantime, I was dying of a liver illness, was obese, depressed and lived in chronic isolation. I couldn't solve my own problems, let alone the ones of the people around me. Even though we can be intelligent, well-educated and driven – that does **NOT** mean that we are ALMIGHTY.

This step is designed to give you a **GOD perspective**. Once you are able to admit your powerlessness, then it is time for you to realize that there **IS a Power Greater than Yourself that CAN solve ALL of the problems you wrote about.**

Here is where a lot of people have problems. They can suspend unbelief for a little while and believe that *'maybe'* there could possibly be a "*Higher Power*" out there. But admit that I am powerless? Never! The problem is that the admission of powerlessness is being viewed as a negative when, in reality, it is a positive. If your car was stuck on a ditch in the middle of nowhere and you had no tools to remove it, what would happen? Do you think that you could use your bare hands to lift the car out of the hole and back on the road?

Or would you need the assistance of somebody else with a truck (*a higher power*) to pull it out. If you sat there day and night refusing to call a truck because that meant you were a loser, would it make any sense? Of course not. Rather, you would admit that you cannot do it on your own and immediately seek for the solution to your problem "*outside of yourself.*" That is what this step is all about. You want to get to a better place in your life. You have goals, petitions and desires that you have put in writing. Now I am asking you to admit that the solution right now is not within you. However, by looking to that Power Greater than Yourself (*the truck*), you <u>CAN</u> find a solution and accomplish your objective.

5) The day **BEFORE** you start the fast, present everything you wrote about in prayer to the God of your understanding. Do it with the internal attitude that **ONLY HE** can remove these problems. Read the list out loud one by one and ask for help. Literally **GIVE ALL OF THEM** to God as you understand Him. Leave nothing out.

Place as much emotion as you can behind the prayer. If you have to scream and yell, so be it. I recall falling on my knees and asking desperately for help as I pounded the wooden floor with my fists and the palms of my hands. I was beaten, hopeless and in dire need of help. And so you, too, have admitted your powerlessness and are in urgent need of supernatural intervention, right? God, in reality, becomes your <u>ONLY</u> hope at this point.

Ask God for protection while you are fasting. Spiritual Warfare can be very real. Ask God to shield you against all evil, darkness and confusion... and ask for the strength to complete the fast. **YOU ARE READY!**

Prayer for Help

Keep the list with you during the fast and add to it as new requests come up. Spend as much time in prayer as you can. This does not necessarily have to be on your knees. If your religious beliefs call for kneeling to pray, by all means do so. I personally believe in kneeling because it reminds me that **I AM NOT ALMIGHTY** and that there is **ONE GREATER** than me. **But do not let yourself be confused or discouraged by religion or dogma**. This is a very personal moment between you and the <u>God of your understanding</u>. Prayer is simply an act of having a conversation with God. You can pray out loud, in your mind or with others. You can pray on your knees, standing up, lying down or standing on your head. <u>God hears you no matter what</u>. If you are new to spirituality, just keep it simple.

One does not have to utter fancy words or extremely long prayers in order to be heard. A simple prayer is just as powerful as any other if it is done with true desire and honesty. **What I want you to understand is this**: When we pray, we are penetrating the invisible world of the Spirit which is

"more real" than the material world. I'll
explain: Look at an object in the room
where you are right now, like a chair. **Do
you see it?** Ok. Where did that chair come
from? **Did it not first exist in a person's
mind?** Yes, it was first invisible, **THEN** its
inventor drew it on paper, then he or she
constructed it and – voila! - it is now part of
our reality for one to see and touch.

So, while fasting, we are focusing our vision
on the invisible world. In prayer, we are
entering **THAT** realm and receiving
supernatural nourishment, healing, comfort
and power. Then we are bringing all of
those great gifts back to **THIS** world.

Spiritual Machine Gun

We are spiritual treasure hunters. And this
treasure is freely-given so that we can share
it with others. The more we share, the more
treasure we receive. This is frequently
referred to the law of Karma. **A question I
am asked regularly is:** What is the
difference between praying versus praying
AND fasting? Big difference. When we pray
but are **NOT** fasting, we are entering the
spirit world with a suitcase to place our

blessings. With fasting, we enter with a super-sized vault! Or, in terms of overcoming addictions and bondage, prayer without fasting gives us a hammer to fight the enemy. With prayer **AND** fasting, we receive a machine gun! See the difference? This does <u>NOT</u> mean, however, that to get powerful results or be heard by God one <u>MUST</u> fast.

But there are times in our lives when circumstances call for fasting as a means of adding high-octane fuel to our prayers.

If you practice a particular religion, continue to do so. Attend those services as you are accustomed to. In addition to prayer, spend time reading spiritual and inspirational books. <u>Important</u>: Carry your fasting journal with you and write regularly about how you are feeling and what is on your mind. You will be surprised how many times the answers we are looking for come as we write! **Remember also that God Uses People.** That is often how he talks to us. What I mean is this: Do **NOT** restrict yourself by thinking that the answers to your prayers can only come through a "*burning bush*" or some other type of supernatural occurrence. While these can and do happen, **I have found that most of us receive our spiritual breakthrough in very subtle ways, often involving others.** So be very sensitive to what is going on around you and do <u>NOT</u> place limits to **HOW God can work things to your benefit.**

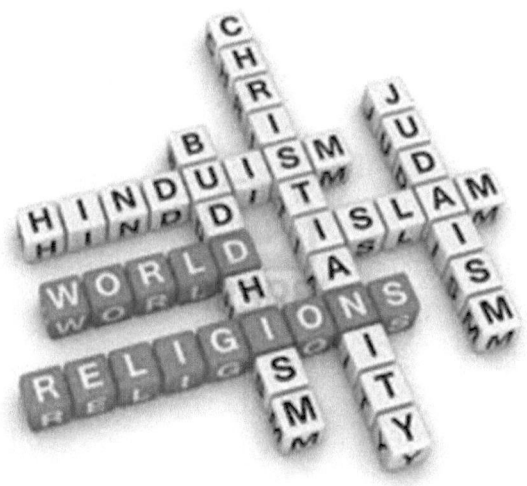

"The World's largest religions have used fasting for thousands of years for many different reasons.

The most common are to attain self-discipline, to receive physical or emotional healing and to receive Divine intervention when in danger or in need of guidance."

Chapter 10:
Fasting & the
World's Religions

At this point I want to take a few moments to talk about fasting from the perspective of Muslims, Christianity and Buddhism. It will be very interesting for you to see the similarities, as well as the different ways in which fasting is practiced. If, like me, you are intrigued by the spiritual power of fasting, then you will enjoy this chapter. In fact, I have received emails from readers who said that they spent most of their time in this chapter, looking up the Bible passages and reading the notes on the other religions.

Fasting has been done for thousands of years. So it behooves us to pay attention to what the past has to share. That way we can maximize the impact of our work together. The greater your understanding of what you are doing, the more faith you will have in your heart to push that internal door that leads to your ultimate dreams.

Fasting in the Bible

* In the Old Testament, the Jews Fasted to seek God's help in threats or times of war (*nation in general*), when loved ones were sick (*David*), in seeking God's forgiveness for themselves and their nation (Ahab, Daniel), and in seeking God's protection and His will (*Ezra*).

Just look up the term, Fasting, in a concordance and observe the abundance of references (*Lev 16:29-31; 23:26-32; Num. 29:7; Psalm 69:10; Acts 27:9*)

* Moses, Elijah, and Jesus all Fasted for 40 days. The Bible records that Spiritual Fasting was not just for the super leaders, rather it was practiced by most, such as during the Judges (*Deut 9:15-18; Jug. 20:26; 1 Kings 21:27*).

(*The Absolute Fasting Moses and The Prophet Elijah did MUST have had divine assistance - Deut. 9:9; 1 Kings 19:8*).

* Israel Fasted at Bethel, in the war against the Benjamites at Mizpah, and in the Philistine war (*Judg. 20:26; 1 Sam 7:6*).

* In the book of Ruth, the Jews Fasted when they heard that Haman had tricked the king into wiping them out (*Esther 4:3-16*).

* David Fasted for Saul and his friend Jonathan, and wept for both his son while he was dying, and for his enemies (*2 Sam. 1:12; 2 Sam. 12:16-23; Psalm 35:11-13*).

* Daniel Fasted for Israel (*Dan. 9:3-5*).

* Fasting accompanied prayer, devotion to God (*Psalm 35:13*), penance (*1 Kings 21:27*), and seeking God earnestly (*2 Sam. 1:12*).

* The effects of Spiritual Fasting with prayer, when it is real and heartfelt, is that it humbles (*Psalm 35:13*), disciplines and corrects wrong behaviors and thinking (Psalm 69:10), and God is more likely to respond to our prayers. (*Ezra 8:21-23*)

* In the New Testament, Spiritual Fasting was practiced when one was faced with temptations (Jesus), in serving God and beginning a new ministry (Antioch), and, when selecting and appointing elders (*Matt. 4:1-2*).

* John the Baptist performed spiritual fasting regularly as a testimony to piety that was real, heartfelt, and pointed to God, not to himself (*Matt. 3:11*).

* Paul listed spiritual fasting among other things that proved he was a minister of Christ (1 Cor. 11:1; 2 Cor. 11:23-28).

* The early church practiced spiritual Fasting as they further sought God's Will, drawing them deeper into His presence (Acts 13:2-3; 14:21-23).

Want more versed? Check these out when you have a chance. If you take the time and read them all, you will find yourself understanding with greater clarity the reason why we are doing this work.

This is not something that I just pulled out of my sleeve. Spiritual fasting is something that has been done for thousands of years by people from all walks of life.

Deuteronomy 9:9-29, 10:1-11; Exodus 34:28; 1 Kings 17:5-7; 2 Chronicles 20:1-29; Esther 4-8; Ezra 8:21-23,31; 10:6, 10:10-11; Daniel 1:8-17; 10:2-3; Joel 1:13-14, 2:12,15,18-27; Matthew 3:4; 4:1-3; Luke 2:36-38; Acts 9:7-19; 10:30-31; 1 Corinthians 7:5; 1 Cor. 7:5; 11:1, 23-28; 2 Col. 2:20-23; 6:4-10; 11:23-28

Fasting and the Quran

The Holy Quran also makes reference to fasting in various places. Here are some that you can also research:

Al-Baqara (The Cow) 2:183 - "O ye who believe! Fasting is prescribed to you as it was prescribed to those before you, that ye may (learn) self-restraint."

Al-Baqara (The Cow) 2:184 - *"(Fasting) for a fixed number of days; but if any of you is ill, or on a journey, the prescribed number (Should be made up) from days later. For those who can do it (With hardship), is a ransom, the feeding of one that is indigent. But he that will give more, of his own free will,- it is better for him. And it is better for you that ye fast, if ye only knew."*

Al-Baqara (The Cow) 2:185 - *"Ramadhan is the (month) in which was sent down the Qur'an, as a guide to mankind, also clear (Signs) for guidance and judgment (Between right and wrong). So every one of you who is present (at his home) during that month should spend it in fasting, but if anyone is ill, or on a journey, the prescribed period (Should be made up) by days later. Allah intends every facility for you; He does not want to put to difficulties. (He wants you) to complete the prescribed period, and to glorify Him in that He has guided you; and perchance ye shall be grateful."*

Al-Baqara (The Cow) 2:187 - *"Permitted to you, on the night of the fasts, is the approach to your wives. They are your garments and ye are their garments. Allah knoweth what ye used to do secretly among yourselves; but He turned to you and forgave you; so now associate with them, and seek what Allah Hath ordained for you, and eat and drink, until the white thread of dawn appear to you distinct from its black thread; then complete your fast Till the night appears; but do not associate with your wives while ye are in retreat in the mosques.*

Those are Limits (set by) Allah. Approach not nigh thereto. Thus doth Allah make clear His Signs to men: that they may learn self-restraint."

Al-Baqara (The Cow) 2:196 - *"And complete the Hajj or 'umra in the service of Allah. But if ye are prevented (From completing it), send an offering for sacrifice, such as ye may find, and do not shave your heads until the offering reaches the place of sacrifice.*

And if any of you is ill, or has an ailment in his scalp, (Necessitating shaving), (He should) in compensation either fast, or feed the poor, or offer sacrifice; and when ye are in peaceful conditions (again), if any one wishes to continue the 'umra on to the hajj, He must make an offering, such as he can afford, but if he cannot afford it, He should fast three days during the hajj and seven days on his return, Making ten days in all.

This is for those whose household is not in (the precincts of) the Sacred Mosque. And fear Allah, and know that Allah Is strict in punishment."

Fasting and Buddhism

In a recent article, Jesuit priest Fr. Thomas Ryan interviewed Rev. Heng Sure, Ph.D. on the Buddhist's perspective on fasting. I am sharing an excerpt of the interview here because I think you will find it very interesting and enlightening. Heng Sure is, director of the Berkeley Buddhist Monastery, president of the Dharma Realm Buddhist Association and senior monastic Bhikshu of the late Chan Master Hsuan Hua. He has been a Buddhist monk in the Chinese Mahayana tradition for 29 years.

"Q: Does fasting hold a very significant place in Buddhist spiritual practice?

A: Fasting in the monastic community is considered an ascetic practice, a "dhutanga" practice. (Dhutanga means "to shake up" or "invigoration.") Dhutangas are a specific list of thirteen practices, four of which pertain to food: eating once a day, eating at one sitting, reducing the amount you eat, on alms-round, eating only the food that you receive at the first seven houses.

These practices are adopted by individuals voluntarily, they are not required in the normal course of a Buddhist monastic's life of practice. The Buddha, as is well known, emphasized moderation, the Middle Way that avoids extremes, in all things. Fasting is an additional method that one can take up, with supervision, for a time.

Q: How did the Buddha's own experience influence the Buddhist approach to fasting?

A: The Buddha's spiritual awakening is directly related to fasting, but from the reverse. That is to say, only after the Buddha stopped fasting did he realize his mahabodhi, or great awakening.

The founding story of the Buddhist faith relates how the Buddha was cultivating the Way in the Himalayas, having left his affluent life as a Prince of India. He sought teachers and investigated a variety of practices in his search for liberation from the suffering of old age, death and rebirth. In the course of his practices he realized that desire was the root of mortality.

He determined, incorrectly, that if he stopped eating he could end desire and gain liberation from suffering. As the story goes, he ate only a grain of rice and a sesame seed per day. Over time he got so thin that he could touch his spine by pressing on his stomach. He no longer had the strength to meditate. He realized that he would die before he understood his mind; further, that desire does not end by force. At that point a young herds maid offered him a meal of milk porridge which he accepted. He regained his strength, renewed his meditation, and realized Buddhahood. So by quitting fasting, and eating in moderation, he realized the central tenet of Buddhist practice, moderation.

Q: For what reasons would Buddhists fast? Would one motivating reason tend to play a more significant role than others?

A: Some Buddhist laity feel that eating low on the food chain creates merit; eating less luxurious food creates an opportunity to serve the planet and all living beings. In this way the dining table becomes a place of practice.

Buddhist monastics who adopt the fasting practice described above do so by and large to purify their bodies and to clarify their thoughts. Fasting allows coarse thoughts to diminish, but strength also diminishes, so there is a trade-off between mental clarity and reduced ability to meditate as long. Some monastics report that the longer they fast, the more strength they have; so not everybody's experience is the same.

The Buddha's own experience showed him that fasting per se did not extinguish desire, it only subdued it. As soon as he resumed eating, his desire returned as well. It took concentration and insight to extinguish desire. The Buddha discovered that desire is rooted in the mind and can be transformed in the mind. Fasting can help that process of transforming desire to wisdom by subduing the body's coarse desires.

Fasting is an aid to the Way, a supplementary practice that can lead to increased mental awareness of the connection between desire and human existence. Moreover fasting highlights one's attachments to food and to good flavor; thus it helps the practitioner to distinguish how much of his or her craving for food is need, and therefore normal and necessary, and how much is greed, and therefore a hindrance to liberation."

Transforming Desire to Wisdom

If you notice, in all of these examples, fasting is always used as a way to receive inner strength and purification from - as the Buddhist monk said - *'coarse'* thoughts. I would say that such list can also include the belief systems and emotions that trigger those thoughts in the first place. I also was very interested in the monk's remark that *"fasting can help that process of transforming desire to wisdom by subduing course desires."* What does that sentence mean to you? **Let's see**: According to the Buddha, it is desire which causes the suffering in human beings. These are truths that he observed while fasting and continued to use when he broke the fast and had his transformation.

Being unhappy because we don't have something we want, or scared because we fear losing something that we cherish.

The Seven Deadly Sins, in essence, are all based on morphed desire. **Pride** is excessive belief in one's own abilities, that interferes with the individual's recognition of the grace of God. It has been called the sin from which all others arise. Pride is also known as **Vanity. Envy** is the desire for others' traits, status, abilities, or situation. **Gluttony** is an inordinate desire to consume more than that which one requires. **Lust** is an inordinate craving for the pleasures of the body. **Anger** is manifested in the individual who spurns love and opts instead for fury. It is also known as wrath. **Greed** is the desire for material wealth or gain, ignoring the realm of the spiritual. It is also called **Avarice or Covetousness. Sloth** is the avoidance of physical or spiritual work.

These all started as natural human instincts; the desire for success, food, companionship, financial security and rest. But somewhere along the line they morphed and became emotional monsters. Soul venom that produces all kinds of painful and destructive behaviors. Why does this happen?

Because of excessive attachment to people, places and things.

Rather than being whole, independent beings, we allow the world around us to control our thoughts, emotions and actions. And so the desire increases, and so its fulfillment continues to slip through our fingers.

Emotional Puppets

Soon we become but puppets, never having personal power of our own. Instead, we are constantly reacting to what is happening on the outside. Reacting with fear, anger, doubt and unbelief because desires *aren't being met as I had hoped.* **This insidious type of mental trap is destructive because it consumes lives**. A man who lives his entire life reacting to the external world is a man who lived his entire life in blindness and nakedness. It is a very subtle yet highly-destructive form of mental/emotional slavery. If my happiness is attached to some person, place, thing, event or whatever... then I am a slave to whatever happens on the outside and cannot have complete peace. People change their minds, and places and things are fleeting and cannot be captured for more than just fleeting moments.

Wisdom, therefore, is the ability to place our thoughts and emotions in their proper perspective so that we can make choices for our lives. Rather than reacting to everything that takes place on the outside, we begin **to accept the fact that we are powerless to control any of them**. Therefore, we can <u>surrender our need to control and start to practice total acceptance</u>. And that acceptance puts an end to the suffering because the need to control has been released and our attachments begin to normalize.

We begin to experience life as healthy individuals. We begin to live our lives fully **WITHOUT** *'needing'* this or that... or collapsing when a person we love is not around for whatever reason.

We can stand on our own in complete peace, **LACKING AND NEEDING NOTHING**. What are your thoughts on this topic? Write about it in your journal. Elaborate on what I said and write how what we are talking about can apply to you. Mediate on the initial part of the famous Serenity Prayer:

"God, grant me the serenity to accept
the Things I cannot change, The
Courage to change the things I can...
And the Wisdom to know the
difference..."

The Buddha and Fasting

What is interesting about the Buddha is
that his moment of enlightenment came
when he 'stopped fasting.' He realized that
all of the fasting in the world would not, in
itself, remove the suffering.

He saw that it was his spiritual
connection with the earth, others and
the universe which made him free. That
he was part of a perfect whole in which
there was no lack, pain or suffering
because this whole was immaterial,
eternal and incorruptible.

And all of this came to him when he
stopped fasting. He did, however, fast. This
begs the question: Did the fasting have
some part in the arrival of this revelation?
Did it help to open the doors within his
mind which allowed him to receive the
enlightenment?

As avid a spiritual seeker as he was, I would venture to say that the answer is <u>definitely yes</u>. What do you think?

The Buddha, as the story tells us, was hungry for spiritual growth <u>above and beyond anything in his life</u>. He left his family, wife, child and all of the luxuries of living in a palace ... he did that **ALL** because he knew in his heart that there had to be more. That there had to be a '*solution*' to human suffering. And finding that solution was the highest calling of his life.

Do you not feel that ending your suffering should be the primary purpose of all that you do?

If we see all that the Buddha accomplished for mankind (*in his lifetime and in the thousands of years since he died*), we know that the answer is yes.

We must find our healing. We must seek it as the most precious thing in this world. Because when we do, <u>the door to new worlds of possibilities will open before your eyes</u>.

And you will wonder where **YOU** have been all along. I hope that you are able to see that, indeed, you are in good company with the practice of spiritual fasting. Take as much time as you need to and internalize, mediate on and write about the examples of fasting that we have looked at in this chapter. One reading is insufficient to gather the fullness of everything that these religions have given us related to fasting for inner healing and liberation.

The Spiritual Virtues

The end result of spiritual renewal and emotional healing is the manifestation of the opposite of the seven deadly sins, the Contrary, Heavenly and Cardinal Virtues, as outlined by the Catholic Church. A while ago we saw a list of symptoms that are usually related to spiritual sickness. We saw how the seven deadly sins started as normal instincts and then morphed as our desire to control got stronger and stronger. Now, however, you are on different footing. You now know that any attempt at controlling people, places and things is a trap designed to keep you unhappy and in pain.

Armed with this new awareness, you can continue to internalize your healing and renewal by starting to manifest virtues rather than sins. Here are virtues which are worthwhile to practice and pursue in our daily lives.

The Cardinal Virtues: Temperance, Justice, Courage, Prudence. Greek philosophers were the first to establish prudence, temperance, courage and justice as virtues.

Later, the Christian Church adopted them and considered them to be of great importance to all of human kind, regardless of religion.

The Theological Virtues: Hope, Faith, Love. The Apostle Paul outlined these chief virtues as being love (*the nature of God*) hope and faith.

The Christian Church called these the three theological virtues because they concluded that man, in his fallen nature, could not attain them. That the virtues could only be received through the act of baptism.

The Seven Contrary Virtues: Humility, Kindness, Abstinence, Chastity, Patience, Diligence, Generosity. **The Contrary Virtues** were derived from the Psychomachia ("*Battle for the Soul*"), an epic poem written by **Prudentius (348-414 A.D.).** These virtues are the exact opposite of the seven deadly sins. They embody positive spiritual power and thus neutralize the seven deadly sins negative pull in the mind and flesh.

Here's how:

Humility destroys Pride
Kindness overcomes Envy
Abstinence heals Gluttony
Chastity (or Purity) vanquishes Lust
Patience wins over Anger
Generosity thwarts Greed
Diligence ends Sloth

The above list is of particular impact to me because it depicts the transition of a human being **from darkness to light.** <u>IT</u> is a picture of me before and after my transformation.

What do you think your life would be like if you constantly were manifesting these virtues?

Let's take a quick look at the list of virtues: prudence, temperance, courage, justice, love, hope, faith, humility, kindness, abstinence, chastity, patience, liberality, diligence, faith, hope, charity, fortitude, justice, temperance and prudence. Here's what I want you to do. **Look up the definition of each and every one of these virtues and write them down in your journal.**

I want each of these to stare at you in black and white whenever you open your notebook. It won't take long at all to do this assignment, but I believe that you will be very gratified with the results. I personally was filled with awe and inspiration when I saw, in simple words, everything that these virtues had to offer me. And, yes... I included the list of virtues in my petitions as outlined in the **Five Steps to Seize the Spiritual Potential of Fasting** that you worked on earlier. Revisit that assignment and expand on it with this new information.

Chapter 11:
The Science of Peace

When it comes to fasting and spiritual growth, there is no greater quality needed than **PATIENCE**. So I want to take a moment to expand my views on this particular virtue so that, when you start the fast, you don't get sacked by the monster of impatience. Human beings are impatient beings by nature. When we don't see results fast enough... when time seems to be crawling, we can become frustrated, negative and unable to hold fast to the vision of what we are working to accomplish.

And that can knock us off track and cause us to lose more precious time rehashing old and self-defeating behaviors. **ENOUGH IS ENOUGH!** The key therefore lies in learning how to handle impatience, frustration and negativity, **WITHOUT** giving in or giving up.

"IF **NOTHING CHANGES, NOTHING CHANGES**".

You might have heard the expression:

"IF WE ALWAYS DO WHAT WE DID, THEN WE WILL ALWAYS GET WHAT WE GOT".

So, if indeed you wish to drop extra pounds, overcome poor eating habits and improve the quality of your life (*what can be more important than this?*), then it is imperative to fine-tune your "<u>patience</u>" muscle. Give it a good workout, make it strong and use it to your advantage.

According to **dictionary.com**, patience means: *"the quality of being patient, as the bearing of provocation, annoyance, misfortune, or pain, without complaint, loss of temper, irritation, or the like. An ability or willingness to suppress restlessness or annoyance when confronted with delay: to have patience with a slow learner. Quiet, steady perseverance; even-tempered care; diligence: to work with patience"*.

I know, I know... patience does not come easy. In fact, it can be quite the challenge, especially when it comes to losing weight, food and eating. Nothing can press our "*impatience*" button as much as the urge to eat. Patience, in essence, is a "*science*". If we look at the word patience in Spanish "*paciencia*", it literally means "*the science of peace*". So, working on patience means learning to remain peaceful (*not overeat, binge or break the fast prematurely*) **IN SPITE** of what is going on in the mind, your body or the events taking place around you.

Of course, when I say "*the body*", I am not saying one should ignore symptoms of illness. You should seek medical care when indicated. I am referring more to the groaning of the belly which is always asking for food and more food.

Dark Night of the Soul

Here are some more virtues that I want you to be aware of because they will greatly strengthen and solidify that all-important patience muscle.

Practice acceptance: We just talked about this in the past chapter in relation to Buddha's revelation. It is so important, that I figured I would mention it again here.

A good friend of mine used to say: *"Robert, it is what it is"*. Although true, I never liked that saying much. At times life will disappoint... we may feel trapped and hopeless. Often, it seems like our cherished goals are taking forever to arrive; we may sometimes even feel that *"nothing will ever happen"*. That is what is called **the dark night of the soul**. No matter how bleak the situation may seem, or how slow everything may *"appear"* to be going, remember that tomorrow may bring the breakthrough you seek. If you give up today, you will never know. It is what it is, but hang on! It is not what happens that matters most, but rather how we react to it. There is a very powerful passage about acceptance in the book **Alcoholics Anonymous** or <u>The Big Book</u> as it is widely known:

"And acceptance is the answer to all my problems today. When I am disturbed, it is because I find some person, place, thing or situation -- some fact of my life -- unacceptable to me, and I can find no serenity until I accept that person, place, thing or situation as being exactly the way it is supposed to be at this moment...

... Nothing, absolutely nothing happens in God's world by mistake. Until I could accept my alcoholism, I could not stay sober; unless I accept life completely on life's terms, I cannot be happy. I need to concentrate not so much on what needs to be changed in the world as on what needs to be changed in me and in my attitudes".

Practice Tolerance: This is what I like to call the art of *"non reaction"*. Practice remaining calm when irritated or provoked. Bear in mind that *"little things affect little minds"*, as said by the **1800s British politician Benjamin Disraeli**. Your ability to remain cool and unflustered when confronted by people, places and things which frustrate you is the <u>best protective shield you can have</u>. It will protect your emotions and help you stay the course, particularly when amidst a long-term fast.

Nothing external can "<u>break</u>" a person. We do it to ourselves. Remember that a lot of us eat because of our emotions. By maintaining poise and composure, you will find strength to keep going when otherwise you might have given up.

Cultivate Faith: Difficulties and frustrations can lead us to give up on our dreams and goals. Faith will help you to grow in maturity and emotional strength. **BELIEVE** that there is an advantage behind every challenge. Stay calm when you are faced with a moment of doubt, anger, fear, etc...

You can use that experience to challenge yourself to stay strong and become closer to God, as you may understand Him. Here is a poem from American Poet **Helen Steiner Rice** that phrases it perfectly:

This Too, Will Pass Away

If I can endure for this minute Whatever is happening to me, No matter how heavy my heart is, Or how dark the moment may be ... If I can remain calm and quiet, With all the world crashing about me, Secure in the knowledge God loves me, When everyone else seems to doubt me ... If I can but keep on believing...

...What I know in my heart to be true, That darkness will fade with the morning, And that "this will pass away, too!" ...Then

nothing in life can defeat me - For as long as this knowledge remains - I can suffer whatever is happening - For I know God will break all the chains - That are binding me tight in "the darkness" And trying to fill me with fear ... For there is "no night without dawning" And I know that "my morning" is near."

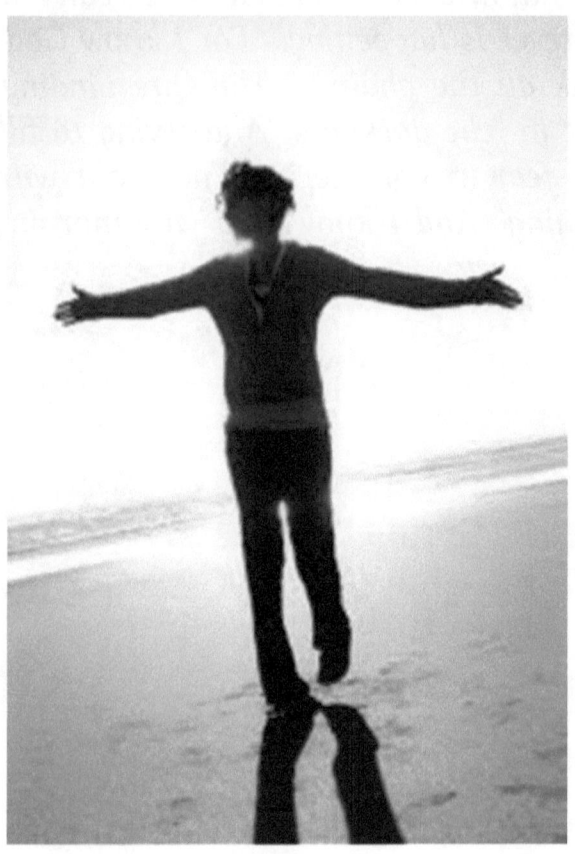

"The garbage will be tossed out, and
you will emerge free; mentally,
physically, spiritually renewed."

Chapter 12:
The Ultimate
Freedom Formula

The time has come to put the pedal to the metal. Here's where you should be right now: You know which type of fast you are going to do and for how long. You have thoroughly completed the **Five Steps to Seize the Spiritual Potential of Fasting.** You have read the chapter on fasting and the world's religions various times and internalized the material. You have become aware that turning desire to wisdom is the key to inner healing and breakthrough.

You have seen how the seven deadly sins can be overcome with seven virtues. You have added the virtues to your fasting petitions as a list of qualities that you want to receive **as replacement of the negative**. Are you with me? Please do not just rush through this material. I want you to take your time and do each individual step to the very best of your ability. **Half measure efforts will yield half measure results.** That isn't what you want, right? So take your time and be thorough.

By the time you reach this section, you should feel pretty comfortable with the material. Now we are going to take more action by adding <u>FIVE</u> more steps to seize the spiritual potential of fasting. These steps will begin with the number 6 because they are a continuation of the five that you've already worked on the chapter "**Seizing the Spiritual Potential.**" When we are done, you will have a total of <u>10 steps </u>to maximize the spiritual benefit of your fast. The first five steps are done **<u>BEFORE</u>** the fast begins. **Steps 6-10**, on the other hand, are designed to be carried out **<u>WHILE</u>** you are fasting. Together, I call these **TEN STEPS** the **Ultimate Freedom Formula**. Ready? Here we go:

6) Personal Inventory: It is time for some in-depth soul searching. Have you ever sat down to write your life story? Not many people have. This can be an extremely powerful way to attain breakthrough and self-realization. However, writing a life inventory **<u>WHILE</u>** fasting is even more powerful.

Why?

Because, when abstaining from food, **we become highly susceptible to introspection and spirituality. This state gives us strength that we don't normally tap into.**

<u>Do this</u>: On the **FIRST** day of the fast (around eight hours after you begin), sit down with your journal to do some work. Make sure that you will be undisturbed during this time. Shut off telephones, TV's and any other gadgets that may distract you. Pray for illumination. **Pray that absolutely everything that is hidden be brought to light**. <u>Start writing</u>. Begin with your earliest memory as a child and talk about people, places and things that surrounded you. Write about what you saw, what was happening and how you felt about it. There doesn't have to be any particular order to the content.

What matters is that you write down in detail everything that you remember. Whatever you struggle with, whatever hurts, whatever limits you (*fear, guilt/shame and feelings of inadequacy, inferiority, failure, bitterness, abandonment, and hopelessness, among other emotional wounds*) – the root causes nearly <u>ALWAYS</u> lie in experiences (*memories*) from childhood, adolescence... all the way to the present. So this step takes you to the very center of your existence. It will unearth many hidden memories, thoughts and feelings that have been standing in your way.

If you have struggled with binging and/or compulsive overeating – *or just a bad diet* -, you may find that food can be closely linked to many painful thoughts, emotions and beliefs. Make sure to write your memories in detail, especially the painful ones. If you recall things you have done that you regret (*ways in which you have injured others*), write them down as well. Put every memory/experience in writing – <u>no matter how uncomfortable</u>. The garbage will be tossed out, and you will emerge free; **mentally, physically, spiritually renewed**. Taking this type of inventory does not have to be time consuming. If you sit uninterrupted and work for one hour daily, there is no reason why you cannot complete the assignment within 72 hours. I'm not saying that you should rush.

Take your time, but be thorough and give yourself completely to the task.

Any time that you have a spare moment – *or when hunger and/or detox symptoms hit hard* – take out the journal and continue with the task. Sometimes it is easy to write. Other times it may be uncomfortable, sometimes <u>very uncomfortable</u>. If you have any *"skeletons in the closet"*, I encourage you to vomit them on paper ... expel that garbage for good. Life is too short to waste, and all of those *"secrets"* only serve to fester and poison the soul.

WE WANT ALL OF THE SMELLY TRASH OUT!

Pray for strength and continue to write. By the time you are done, you will have written the history of your life. It is absolutely imperative that you leave nothing out. It doesn't matter how tasteless it may be, you **<u>MUST</u>** get it out of you and put it in writing. If it is embarrassing, then so be it. Like my friend John says:

"You can't save your face and your ass at the same time." :-)

Once you feel **COMPLETELY SATISFIED** that you have covered **ABSOLUTELY EVERYTHING**, then you are ready to move to the next step.

7) Disclosure: Toward the beginning of this book, I mentioned to you that you were going to need the support of **ONE** person that you trusted. Somebody that you are close to but not related to. If you have a best friend, then that would be the best option. It is now time to take the next step in the housecleaning, which is **DISCLOSING** to another human being everything that you have written in your life inventory. This is nothing new. Catholicism, for example, has practiced the discipline of confession for centuries. In many ways that is exactly what you are doing. You are *"confessing"* (telling another person) about your past **with the aim of being free of it.** It is possible that you may suddenly start to feel a lot of resistance to taking this step.

You may get angry, want to punch me out or just dismiss the step as ridiculous, something left for priests and nuns, a stupid request, an unacceptable breach of privacy and on and on. Those feelings are normal.

Once the emotional cancer is exposed, it will fight for its 'survival' by causing you to reject the very steps that are leading you toward healing. You certainly won't be trumpeting all of this information from the rooftops. You are simply dumping it with ONE person that you trust, who will preserve your privacy and never divulge what was said. IF, however, you feel that there is nobody around you that you trust with the information, then you can go to the nearest Catholic church and ask a priest to listen to your inventory. You don't have to be Catholic to talk to a priest. Most are happy to help. Whatever you decide to do, do it at once and take the action.

Do this: **AFTER** you have completed the life inventory, call your friend and make an appointment to sit together undisturbed for two to three hours. Make sure that this meeting take place no longer than two days after you complete the inventory. You don't stock trash in your house, do you? Of course not. Garbage stinks and it is promptly removed from the home and dumped in the trash bin where it belongs. Likewise, these painful memories and experiences that you have written about need to be thrown out. If you procrastinate, you will defeat the whole purpose. We want to strike while the iron is hot! Tell your friend that you've been doing some serious housecleaning and soul-searching. Tell him/her that part of this process requires disclosure of every detail of your past to someone, and that you need his/her help. All you want is someone to listen, that's all. **No comments or opinions are needed**. Only a person who is willing to listen as you carry out this liberating task.

The objective here is to release, get rid of, and be done with shame, fear, guilt, secrets, and anything else that bothers you, causes you to feel less than or bad about yourself.

Releasing these feelings will greatly cut down on emotional eating. Once written on paper, the next step is to open our mouths and get it out. It is a straightforward but effective way to achieve breakthrough and tap into immense spiritual healing. We simply tell the truth about ourselves to ourselves, to another person, and to God in **an attitude of self- responsibility, acceptance, and forgiveness.**

Recovery groups like **Alcoholics Anonymous, Narcotics Anonymous and Gamblers Anonymous** utilize this simple act of confession as a vital step in the recovery from those respective addictions. Bottom line: IT **WORKS!**

8) Willingness To Let Go: Once you have finished Step 7 and left your friend, find a place where you can be alone for a while. If you truly gave yourself to this assignment, then you have done **A LOT!** Sit in silence and meditate on what you just did. Write your thoughts and feelings on the journal. Were you thorough in disclosing everything? Is there anything that you forgot? If you suddenly remember some event that was not written in the journal, write it down. Later on, when you talk to your friend again, take him or her aside and disclose that particular event.

Repeat this process anytime something else comes up. Once the top is taken out, many memories may begin to flush out over a period of weeks and months. Simply write down what you remembered, call your friend and disclose. All in all, doing an honest and thorough Step 7 wipes the slate clean. Now it is time to call upon the God of your understanding and ask Him to eradicate **EVERYTHING** that has harmed and/or limited you. Remember, the old way is what got us here.

Are you ready to let go of the old? Are you prepared to release the former ways of thinking and behaving in favor of a better way? There is always room for improvement in our lives.

So, yes, this applies to you **EVEN** if you don't feel you have much you need to change. **This step is about desire for a better life/health and the willingness to do whatever it takes to achieve AND maintain it.** Our spirituality has to be practical and based on action.

9) **Prayer:** Now it is time to **LET GO OF THE PAST**. We do this through prayer, giving **ALL** of our past to the God of our understanding and asking Him to cleanse and heal our souls... asking Him to **wipe out everything that stands in the way of us living our life to its highest potential**. When you are prepared, you may like to say something like this:

"My Creator, I now give YOU my mind, body and spirit. I give YOU all of my past and all that has hurt and limited me. I ask YOU, by YOUR Grace, to heal my entire being, to purge my mind and emotions from all that has harmed me. Let YOUR joy and peace overflow from my heart. Set me free from the past... fill me with YOUR light, power and strength. Renew me, refresh me... grant me YOUR liberty and YOUR vision for my life, that I may be of maximum use to YOU and to my fellow man. From this day forward, I live in YOUR shadow and YOUR might. I now believe this has been done and receive the complete transformation YOU have now given me... Amen".

Of course, the wording is optional... but you get the idea. What matters is that you **do this with all of your heart.** This is not a religious type of prayer. Whatever comes out of your mouth will suffice if you truly mean it. Spend as much time as you need to in prayer. Put your heart into it and realize that this is YOUR life. At this time, a sense of great peace will come over the soul. I have seen people attain amazing spiritual awakenings. Many are healed of physical disease and life-long mental barriers.

Just sit in silence and savor the moment. Spend as much time alone as you need, and keep writing in your journal as you are moved to do so.

10) Commit to Continue Exploring Your Spiritually: Having completed all of these steps and finished your work, continue the fast until you reach the number of days that you had decided to so. Each day, take out this book and read the prayer above. Do it in the mornings at the time that you would usually have breakfast. Read the prayer at least three times daily, and continue to write in your journal as much as possible. In addition, it is time for you to make a commitment with yourself that you are going to continue to explore and nourish your spirituality for the rest of your life.

Spiritual growth and development is not a goal; it is a **lifelong journey that requires time, energy and dedication**. I have seen people attain amazing spiritual awakenings through prayer and fasting. Many are healed of physical disease and life-long mental barriers. However, when the novelty of the spiritual *"high"* wears off, one is often tempted to give up.

Please write in your journal some of the actions that you can take **AFTER** the fast to continue your spiritual path. This can include: returning to your accustomed religious services, learning about the different global religions, doing daily devotionals, spending time daily in prayer/meditation, getting involved in some type of charitable service, among many others. If you have not been very spiritual, any small step in that direction will help.

Chapter 13:
Signs of Spiritual Growth

Remember: Steps 1-5 are done <u>BEFORE</u> the fast. Steps 6-10 are carried out <u>WHILE</u> fasting. The emphasis is on the combination of fasting <u>PLUS</u> internal housecleaning and prayer. At this point many readers ask me: "*Robert, how do I know if these steps are really working in my life?*" Indeed, that is a hard question to answer because we are each so different. However, there are some general personality traits that indicate spiritual awakening/growth. Here are some of the most common:

1. Self Control: A spiritually committed person throws out bad habits that offer temporary pleasure (*before ultimately bringing suffering*) and instead chooses the lasting satisfaction of emotional health found through self-control. Many people turn to alcohol, drugs, gambling and compulsive overeating to cope with anxiety and unpleasant memories, but this sort of avoidance keeps us from acquiring the <u>inherent soul wisdom</u> needed to overcome trials and be lastingly happy.

2. Humility: A spiritual awakening is cultivated by caring about the well-being of others and contributing to life <u>WITHOUT</u> the desire for recognition. Rather than taking credit for good actions from an egotistical perspective, a person on a spiritual path presents successes as **offerings to the God of his/her understanding - emphasizing gratitude rather than pride.**

3. Calmness and Concentration: If one compared God's presence to the bottom of a lake, it would only be visible when the ripples of *"constant thought"* subsided and the water became calm. If the water is muddy or disturbed (*endless thought, worry*), the bottom (*God's presence*) cannot be seen. Events, memories, concerns, and desires all try to intrude incessantly throughout our day. A person who is spiritually-awake tends to handle these daily pressures with greater calmness, <u>focusing his/her mental energy on solutions rather than problems</u>.

4. Non-attachment: Part of spiritual awakening is mental freedom from possessions. By practicing non-attachment, one can enjoy things and perform material duties with a sense of service rather than personal gain. The ego wants to cling to objects, ideas, youth, money, power and other aspects of worldly experience; by letting go of these things gracefully when they have served their time, inner peace is strengthened.

5. Intuition: Intuition is a dependable source of wisdom and guidance to one who is receptive to its subtle advice. When one taps into this resource by surrender and daily meditation, one is able to hear and trust what the right course of action is to fulfill his/her best interests.

6. Self-Knowledge: By being aware in each present moment of one's thoughts, intentions, and desires, one can begin to chisel away unwanted personal qualities and, instead, reinforce new traits that lead to triumph over negativity.

7. Freedom: In the end, one is individually responsible for his/her own habits, mistakes, and resolutions. Once contact is made with the God of our understanding, however, we tap into a source of power that gives us <u>TRUE</u> freedom. Life takes on a deeper, richer meaning than that of simply satisfying our immediate cravings and/or succumbing to a painful habit and/or addiction. Obsessions leave us. We come to realize that this new spiritual strength is helping us to do what we could not do in the past.

We all make mistakes and sometimes get off track. But we get up, dust ourselves off and get right back on the saddle. It's all about progress. So, when doing steps 6-10 of the **Ultimate Freedom Formula**, be tough on yourself - **but do it with compassion**! I have yet to find a single person who, following these steps to the best of his/her ability, does not notice a change – *often a dramatic one* – in his/her life. Now it is your turn! Open your mind and heart; set aside your doubts and fears. This is the journey into the center of your being. May the powerful light of the Spirit guide you into the breakthrough you've been waiting for!

Chapter 14:
Bringing it All Together

1) Decide Which Method of Fasting You Are Going to Use and For How Long You Will Fast: As I suggested, 7-10 days is optimal for the purposes of this work. Get in touch with your heart and let intuition guide you into the perfect time frame. Push yourself. Shoot for 21 days if possible. Believe me, you won't regret it. Whatever temporary discomfort you go through will be nothing in comparison to the huge benefits that you will gain mentally, physically and spiritually.

2) Mark your calendar and decide specifically <u>when</u> you will be fasting. It is best to start at a time when you don't have that many activities like, for example, the weekend. Sunday is always a good start day. If you are able to take some time off to do this work, do so. If not, don't worry. You can still do it. Most of us cannot just stop our daily schedule in that fashion. Regardless of what your situation may be, make the decision and mark the calendar. Done!

3) **Spend time in your journal going through the Five Steps to Seize The Spiritual Potential of Fasting.** As you recall, those <u>initial five steps</u> represent the 'pre-fasting' part of your housecleaning. Make sure that you have answered all of the questions thoroughly and that every single petition and prayer request is listed. Don't forget to add the list of virtues that we discussed. You will definitely want to place those in the list of qualities that you want for yourself. Remember that your healing will happen **so that you can then share your light with others who still suffer.**

4) **Get All of The Supplies Needed For the Fast.** If you have decided to water fast, make sure to have plenty of good water to drink, as well as seltzer water (*sparkling water/club soda*) and green tea. Green tea has body-heating properties that will help to soothe hunger as well as give you energy. Seltzer water is another handy fasting tool that I use to quiet hunger pangs and detox symptoms. You also can purchase chamomile tea and have a cup at night before you turn in. If you are doing a juice fast, then you need to purchase the fruit and veggie juice. You have already marked your

calendar and selected a start date. Make sure to have all of the supplies in place **the day before you begin the fast.**

5) Speak to the person you have chosen to act as your support and let him or her know when you are planning to start the fast. Make an appointment to see him or her around the **FOURTH** day of your fast. That day, you two will have a long chat, and the course of your life could very well be transformed forever. Tell him/her that you will need his/her support more than ever, and that you need to have a sit down. Tell him/her that you will need at least three hours of his/her time and arrive at a date and time. This date and time, of course, is contingent on your completion of the life inventory. So setting the appointment can be a good way to *"pressure yourself"* into following through.

6) On the **FIRST** day of the fast, after around 8 hours of fasting, roll up your sleeves and get to work on the life inventory. Make sure that to wait until you have been fasting for at least those 8 hours. By then, you will be feeling the sting of abstinence. The spirit-focus that we have talked about will come into play. Make absolutely certain that you know what you are supposed to do. If your mind tells you that all this business of writing an inventory is silly/hogwash, just tell it to shut up and... do it anyway! I went through the same resistance and can tell you that I am **VERY** glad that I did not give in to the doubt and scorn. It's all in your hands now. By Day 4, the inventory should be completed and you will be ready to sit down and empty all of that trash out of your soul and out of your life once and for all.

7) Once you have thoroughly disclosed every nick and cranny of the past to your friend, retire to a private place. Spend time thinking about what you have done, writing down anything that you may have forgotten (*for later disclosure*).

When you are ready, refer to the final prayer and say it with all of your heart. Enjoy the divine peace that comes. Some people choose to take the pages of the journal and burn them... a symbolic action geared to impress upon your soul that all of that trash has been wiped out, <u>NEVER</u> to return again.

8) Refer to the spiritual growth list. Make a firm determination within yourself to continue growing spiritually. Take concrete steps in that direction as, for example, starting a daily time of prayer and meditation. You are walking on a new road now, my friend. But you must remain vigilant and work to maintain your freedom. Doing another fast in three months' time putting together a follow-up life inventory is highly recommended. For instructions on how to break the fast, visit that specific page at the main website **FitnessThroughFasting.com.**

God bless,

ROBERT DAVE JOHNSTON

Grab The Entire Collection:

Volume 1: The 'Permanent Weight Loss' Diet

Volume 2: The Intermittent Fasting Weight Loss Formula

Volume 3: How to Lose 30 Pounds (Or More) In 30 Days with Juice Fasting

Volume 4: Lose The Belly Fat Fast, And For Good!

Volume 5: Lose the Emotional Baggage: Transform Your Mind & Spirit with Fasting

Volume 6: How to Break a Fast (or Diet) and Keep the Weight Off

Volume 7: Compilation Volumes 1-6 -> Get All 5 For The Price Of 3!

Also by Robert Dave Johnston:

How to Lose Weight & Keep it Off by Transforming the Mind & Behaviors

Volume 1: How to Build a Rock-Solid Foundation That Supports Long-Term Weight Loss

Volume 2: How to Lose Weight & Keep it Off By Reprogramming The Subconscious Mind

Volume 3: How to Beat Diet Hunger and Junk Food Cravings

Volume 4: How to Escape the Diet "Time Trap" and Succeed in Weight Loss

Volume 5: How to Cheat on Your Diet (And Get Away With It)

Volume 6, Compilation: All 5 for the Price Of 3

Also By Robert Dave Johnston:

Detoxify Your Body, Lose Weight, Get Healthy & Transform Your Life

Volume 1- The 10-Day 'At Home' Colon Cleansing Formula

Volume 2- The 30-Day Kidney, Parasite & Liver Detox Weight Loss Method

Volume 3- Lose Weight Fast & Detoxify With Intermittent Fasting & At-Home Coffee Enemas

Volume 4 - Compilation: Get All 3 For The Price Of 2! Detoxify Your Body, Lose Weight, Get Healthy & Transform Your Life - Volumes 1-3

Don't forget to check the articles and growing health community at: FitnessThroughFasting.com